The Adrenal Reset Cookbook: Recipes That Balance Hormones and Help You Lose Weight Quickly and Safely

Table of Contents

RECIPES FOR ADRENAL TYPES

Asian Flank Steak

Ingredients:

- 8 oz. Flank Stead
- 1 tsp vegetable oil
- 1 C sliced peppers

MARINADE:

- 2 tsp soy sauce
- 1 tsp cornstarch
- 1 C fresh ginger
- 2 C sliced onion
- 1 teaspoon red wine

Directions:

1. This is a really simple recipe.
2. The steak you will cut into strips and cook in the skillet with the oil and cook on both side, once brown, add the peppers and sauté with the steak and set aside.
3. Mix the sauce ingredients in a bowl and add steak to marinade (before cooking over skillet).
4. Eat with lettuce or tortilla shells

Chicken Vegetable Soup

Ingredients:

- 1 Chicken, cut up
- 3 C diced celery
- 3 C carrots diced
- 8 oz. chicken broth

Directions:

1. If you want to cook this in the slow cooker, add chicken and broth to slow cooker.
2. Set on low for 4-6 hours, after that time, add vegetables and cook for another 1-2 hours on low or simmer.
3. Great family meal or can be divided up and frozen for frequent meals.

Sole Provençal

Ingredients:

- 1 lbs. sole
- 1 tsp. olive oil
- 1 T minced garlic
- 1can diced tomatoes, sliced
- ¼ lbs. diced mushrooms

Directions:

1. Start with preheating your oven to 400 degrees and while this is heating up, you will want to take your skillet and heat or sauté your mushrooms and your other vegetables on stovetop for 50 minutes.
2. Cut up the fish and add to baking dish, add sauté vegetables, and bake for 15-20 minutes.

Red Snapper "Scallops"

Ingredients:

- 8 oz. frozen snapper
- 1 tsp. olive oil
- 1 T white wine
- 1 T water
- 1 lime cut up, or juiced
- 1 T cilantro

Directions:

1. Sauté the fish over a skillet on medium heat with the olive oil and cut up lime or squirt juice over the snapper.
2. Add fresh cilantro over the fish and enjoy.

Chicken Burgers

Ingredients:

- 1 lbs. ground turkey
- 2 T dried breadcrumbs
- ½ C minced onions
- ½ C chopped onions
- 1 egg, beaten
- 1 tsp. vegetable oil

Directions:

1. Add ground turkey and everything but the oil to a mixing bowl and blend well.
2. Make patties and cook on skillet with the vegetable oil.
3. Serves four.

Turkey bobs

Ingredients:

- 6 lbs. turkey meat
- ¼ C soy sauce
- ¼ C dry sherry
- 1 T fresh ginger
- 1 tsp vinaigrette
- ½ tsp. red pepper flakes
- ½ C minced garlic

Directions:

1. This is really simple and fun to make.
2. Mix everything together and add the turkey to the skewers and add to the grill, oven or stove top.

Fruit Ice

Ingredients:

- 1 lbs. choice of your fruit
- ⅛ C sugar
- 1 envelope unflavored gelatin
- ¼ C lemon juice

Directions:

1. Sprinkle gelatin over lemon juice, let stand.
2. In a small pan, combine sugar with 1 cup of water.
3. Stir over low heat until sugar dissolves; bring to boil and boil gently, uncovered and without stirring, five minutes.
4. Remove from heat.
5. Add the gelatin and stir until dissolved.
6. Puree the fruit in a blender until smooth, and add gelatin mixture to it; blend until smooth.
7. Turn into an 8" X 2" pan.
8. Freeze about 2 hours.
9. Turn into a chilled bowl and beat quickly with a mixer or rotary beater until smooth but not melted.
10. Return to the pan and freeze several hours, until firm.

Chocolate Cookies

Ingredients:

- 3 egg whites
- 6 squares unsweetened chocolate
- ½ tsp vanilla extract
- ½ C sugar

Directions:

1. Set oven to 350 degrees, and mix ingredients, and spoon batter onto greased cookie sheet, bake for 12-15 minutes.

Sample Meal Plans

BREAKFAST:

1 cup of hot whole-grain cereal with

½ cup of skim milk Coffee or tea (with a teaspoon of sugar if desired)

LUNCH:

A large green salad with clear diet dressing (see recipe section)

3 ounces of water-packed tuna Steamed green beans

1 slice of French bread

½ cantaloupe

Coffee, tea, or parsley tea (with a small amount of sugar or honey if desired)

DINNER:

4 ounces broiled steak (or you may substitute poultry, fish, or legumes)

½ cup of bulgur wheat (see recipe section)

Steamed zucchini

1 glass of skim milk

1 piece of fruit

Parsley tea (with a teaspoon of sugar if desired)

BREAKFAST:

1 cup of hot whole-grain cereal with

½ cup of skim milk Coffee or tea (with a teaspoon of sugar if desired)

<u>LUNCH</u>:

A large green salad with clear diet dressing (see recipe section)

3 ounces of water-packed tuna

Steamed green beans

1 slice of French bread

½ cantaloupe Coffee, tea, or parsley tea (with a small amount of sugar or honey if desired

<u>DINNER</u>:

Ingredients:

- 4 ounces broiled steak (or you may substitute poultry, fish, or legumes)
- ½ cup of bulgur wheat (see recipe section)
- Steamed zucchini
- 1 glass of skim milk
- 1 piece of fruit
- Parsley tea (with a teaspoon of sugar if desired)

Day One

BREAKFAST:

½ C Cottage Cheese and Water

LUNCH:

Spinach Salad with one can water tuna, side of peaches and tea or water

DINNER:

Flank Steak stir Fry with salad, any vegetable with tea water or lemonade

Day Two

BREAKFAST:

1 container (6 oz.) yogurt

LUNCH:

Large Taco salad, clear dressing

Side fruit salad

Tea or water

DINNER:

Red Snapper recipe above

Side salad

Tea or Water

Day Three

BREAKFAST:

1 C cereal with skim milk

LUNCH:

1 C grapes

Side salad

Tea or lemonade

DINNER:

Chicken burgers, no bun (optional)

1 C fruit of your choice

Side salad

Water

Day Four

BREAKFAST:

1 C oatmeal

LUNCH:

Baked potato

1 piece of fruit

DINNER:

Turkey Kabobs

1 C fruit

Cookies (see recipe above)

Tea or water

Day Five

<u>BREAKFAST</u>:

½ C cottage cheese and strawberries (sliced)

<u>LUNCH</u>:

A large green salad with clear diet dressing (see recipe section)

3 ounces of mozzarella cheese toasted on

1 slice of whole-grain bread Steamed spinach

1 cup of fresh cherries iced tea or parsley tea (with a teaspoon of sugar if desired)

<u>DINNER</u>

Chicken Soup

Side salad, clear dressing

Water

Change it up a little with these alternatives:

Morning alternatives

Yogurt of your choice

½ C cottage cheese

1 C cereal

Coffee, tea, or parsley tea (with a small amount of sugar or honey if desired)

Wait 4 hours

Lunch alternatives

Salad: taco, Mediterranean, fruit

Olive oil, coconut oil, apple vinegar, coconut oil

1 C grain, or 1 piece of bread (gluten free is best)

Water or tea

WAIT 6 hours before next meal

Evening alternatives

Your choice of 4 oz. meat or legumes

A serving of grain, your choice, whole or refined (but give preference to whole grains such as brown rice, whole wheat, or whole-grain pasta).

As at lunch, a serving is ½ cup. Steamed vegetables, your choice, as much as you like.

2 teaspoons of vegetable oil (you may use it in preparation of the poultry, fish, or eggs, or on the vegetables).

Milk, tea or water

Choice of the same fruits as for lunch OR 2 chocolate cookies OR fruit ice (see recipe section).